WILLOW SOWLE

THE NEW DR. NOWZARADAN DIET PLAN AND COOKBOOK FOR BEGINNERS

A Beginner's Guide to Healthy Weight Loss with Dr. Nowzaradan's Proven Diet Plan (2024)

Contents

INTRODUCTION

Finding a surgeon, receiving surgery approval, and then undergoing the procedure are just the beginning of the process to lose weight. It can be quite difficult for many people to form healthy new habits and give up bad old ones. Making these changes does get easier with time, but you will need to learn to deal with stress and daily problems without turning to food.

If you've never worked out, you could be pleasantly pleased to discover that you like the activity and the stress-relieving benefits that come with it. Your hectic life may benefit in a number of ways if you set aside an hour each day for exercise.

Limiting your daily calorie intake is not sufficient. Numerous parts of your life will need to alter, including the way you approach eating, prepare meals, and even how you dress.

Your success depends on you being able to rely on friends, family, and even other people who have undergone weight loss surgery. A crucial step in the process is to find someone who will listen to you or who can relate to what you are going through.

It is reasonable to say that after surgery, your life will change significantly, most of the time for the better. As your body gets smaller, you'll feel better, look better, have more energy, and be far healthier than you ever thought possible. The next time you go grocery shopping, grab a sack of potatoes, and see how long it takes for your arms to get fatigued if you have any doubts about how much better you will feel after losing weight. Losing that weight repeatedly and no longer having to lug those additional pounds along with you will feel wonderful.

All of these improvements require work, but the benefits are well worth the effort. A few benefits of losing weight include being able to wear smaller clothing, boosting your confidence, and going for a walk or up a flight of stairs without feeling weary. Even while weight loss surgery won't solve all of your problems, it could be able to eliminate some of them, including type 2 diabetes, high blood pressure, and sleep apnea.

As you lose weight, things you might have avoided in the past will become much easier to obtain. Imagine going to the movies and being able to relax in your seat or taking a vacation to a warm beach and feeling at ease while wearing a swimming suit. As you work towards your weight loss objective, you will also be achieving other goals, like being able to run and play with your kids or effortlessly going from one end of the mall to the other.

CHAPTER 1: THE 1200-CALORIE DIET

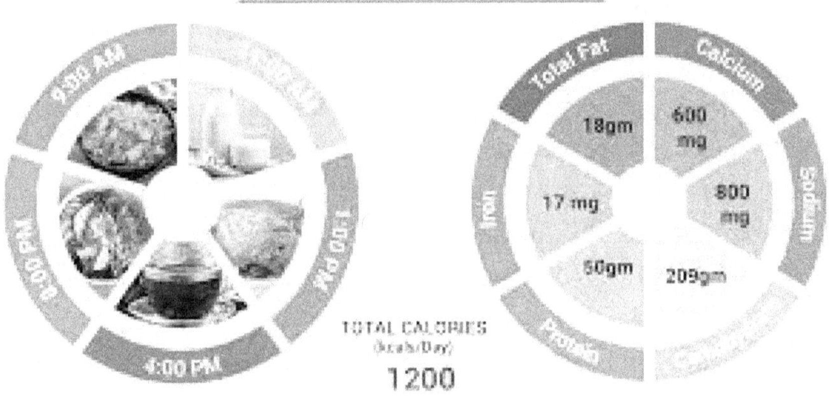

It is a diet regimen that promises to cure people of their most serious medical issues. All of your meals will now, for the first time, be prepared per the 1200-calorie diet. Just a few straightforward, amusing, and healthful ingredients make up its ingredients list:

Replace highly addictive and unhealthy foods, and abstain from alcohol, smoking, and tobacco use both before and after surgery. Get rid of your typical diet of fatty and sugary meals and switch to something delicious and nutritious in their stead.

Why choose a 1200-calorie recipe right now? Avoid needless, expensive surgery for obesity.

Here, for a fraction of the cost, is the nicest, healthiest, and only long-term option. Even after weight loss surgery, you are still allowed to eat 1200 calories each day. Live among your loved ones without feeling alien.

You may prepare scrumptious meals on your own that are healthy.

You can eat with perfect confidence that YOUR diet is secure and wholesome. Make tasty, wholesome, and simple meals.

The patient's health suffers as a result of the other diets, which are both costly and risky. The diet that is promoted on television will not only deprive you of all rights, but it will also seriously harm your health.

The customized smoothie that makes up the diet's major component is made up of the following ingredients:

Lacking in sugar, oil, and fat very low cholesterol levels. lacks salt.

a lot of protein.

High in magnesium, potassium, and calcium, which are commonly useful in lowering cholesterol, body fat, and blood pressure.

You won't need any artificial colors or flavors anymore because the ingredients combine to offer remarkable health advantages. Boost your happiness, general health, and looks.

Homework can be done there. Making your diet is simple.

Only if you do it will it be effective.

The 1200-calorie diet is a customized eating regimen that was created to not only assist you in losing weight but also serve as a great alternative to weight reduction surgery. Without any negative effects, it encourages eating less than 1200 calories per day.

The creation and adherence to a diet consisting of 1200 calories are advised by doctors for overweight and obese people. You will have complete control over your diet because it was created by you.

However, people who desire to shed only a few pounds and then quit should not follow the 1,200- calorie diet plan. Patients who want to permanently eliminate extra weight and its associated hazards may consider it.

CHAPTER 2: ADOPTING A 1200-CALORIE DIET

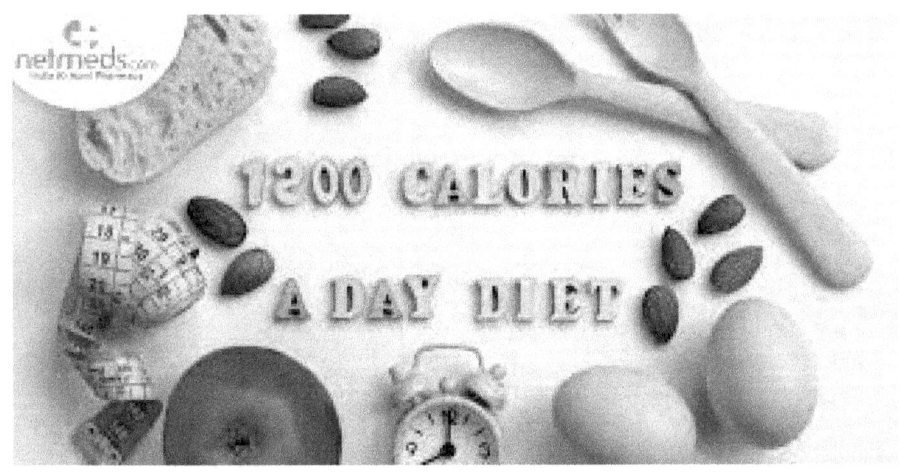

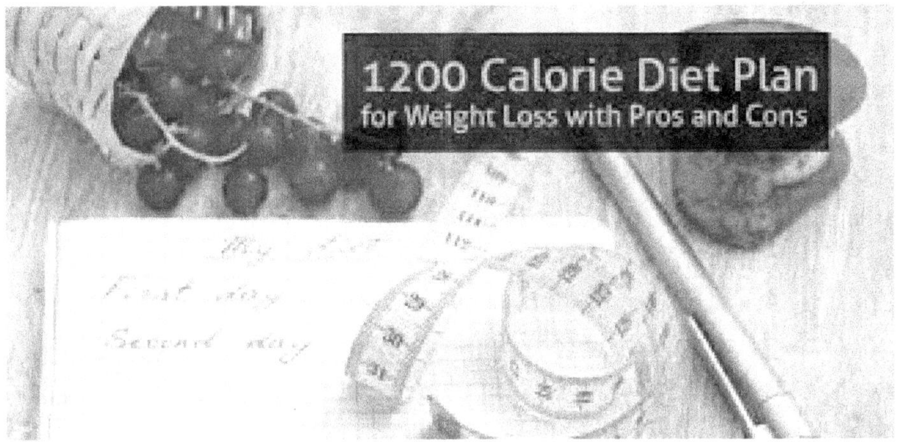

In the 1200-calorie diet, there are no tags. The fundamental plan is simple and uncomplicated. You must consume a total of less than or equal to 1,200 calories per day to adhere to the requirements of the diet.

Some of the applications that can truly help you keep track of how many calories you eat include Muffin Top, Lose It, Cron-o-meter, FatSecret, and SparkPeople.

Setting a weight goal for yourself is key, as is being careful to prevent losing muscle mass when losing weight, as the diet is more important for weight loss than for weight maintenance. After you reach your target weight, you have the choice of increasing your calorie intake, but you should continue to follow a healthy diet plan to keep your weight under control.

I must tell you that if you decide to follow this diet, you will probably eat fewer calories each day than you might imagine if you're used to consuming a lot of calories. This is a result of the possibility that taking the supplement could force your body to experience hunger. Another justification for consulting a doctor before beginning a diet is the potential risk to your health.

Eating meals that are healthy and will keep you feeling full for a long period is crucial to fending off the hunger pangs that are common when dieting. To sate your hunger, consume a small amount of nourishing meals.

Among the countless options, some healthy meals to try include watermelon, salad, grapefruit, vegetables, and fruits with a high water content.

You are allowed to eat six times a day with snacks in between those meals under the plan, as well as between each of your three meals. Additionally, you'll be able to engage in less strenuous activities, aiding you in your effort to lose weight.

When adhering to this diet plan, make sure your 1200-calorie meal plan includes a selection of healthy and well-balanced meals. To avoid nutritional shortages and to guarantee that you regularly consume enough water to stay hydrated and control your hunger, you must do this.

What to Remember About Cereals High-fiber, nutrient-dense grains to include in your diet include whole wheat, millet, ragi, amaranth, oats, and barley. Make your meals more varied by using these various flours. Instead of refined, sugar-coated, rose-flavored cereal, breakfast would be better served with a bowl of multigrain cereal. It doesn't imply that you shouldn't eat refined grains; rather, it suggests that you should only do so sometimes.

Idlu, Doa, and Uttaram are three varieties of polished rice that are excellent choices for a substitute in a balanced diet. Replace it with rocket and add a lot of raw vegetables to white bread to make a high-fiber salad.

These are necessary for our bodies ability to develop, heal, and maintain themselves, as well as for our hormones, blood, and immune systems. You might consume less cereal if you eat meals that include at least one form of protein.

Vegetable sources of protein include dal, besan, ou, ranger, and see. In comparison to beef, organ meats, and pig, chicken, fish, and eggs are the healthiest non-vegetarian protein sources, in that order. Choose lower-calorie alternatives to paneer and cheese, which are both rich in fat calories.

Fats: They are essential and shouldn't be cut out of your diet. You can reduce the number of calories you eat by limiting how much food you eat, and you can do this without compromising taste or any of the positive health effects that come with it.

Even while refined vegetable oils are beneficial, you shouldn't limit yourself to a single type. Vegetable oil has the same number of calories and fat as ghee and clarified butter, however, the saturated fat level of ghee and clarified butter is higher. It's okay to take one TR every day.

Vegetables: Finally, a dish that will completely quench your appetite. Hungry? Eat a carrot for a warm, salty snack. You may also boil your vegetables, blend them, and make soup from them. You can also juice your vegetables for a cool, refreshing beverage. There should be three servings each day.

Every other vegetable serving weighs 100 grams, whereas a serving of leafy vegetables weighs 150 grams.

However, since you are permitted to consume as much food as you choose, you don't need to worry about your weight. Sweet potatoes, potatoes, and other root and tuber foods are permitted in the stash only.

They are actually and truly capable of giving you the same number of calories as their contribution to the meal.

Fruit: This stuff makes a great dessert. Take two portions of 100–150 grams of mango and banana (when in season).

Milk and items made with milk: There should be milk at every meal, whether it be skim milk, fat-free dahi, or skim milk ricotta. Ricotta prepared from skim milk is another option. A ruddling of fat-free milk may satisfy a late-night craving for anything sweet.

Make sure you are not in any way depriving yourself of the flavor of food, regardless of how many calories you intend to consume. Try new foods, eat your meals whole, and follow the seasons.

Not only can maintaining your health help you keep your current weight, but it will also give you a glowing complexion and plenty of energy.

Chapter 3: CAN IT AID IN WEIGHT LOSS?

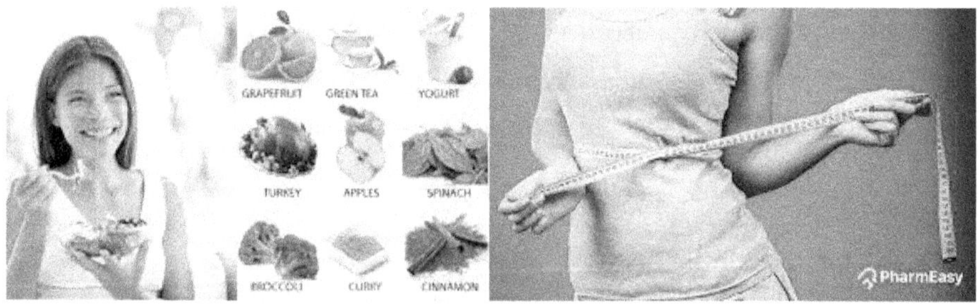

The creation of a calorie deficit is required for successful weight loss. Some medical professionals assert that reducing daily caloric intake by 500 to 750

calories is the most effective strategy for short-term weight loss. In a separate study, adults were assigned one of three weight-loss regimens: 500 calories per day, 1,200–1,500 calories per day, or 1,500–1,800 calories per day. Those who adhered to a 1,200– 1,500-calorie-per-day diet for one year lost an average of 15 pounds (6.8 kg). In contrast, 23 percent of the 4,588 participants who were consuming a 1,200-calorie diet bowed out of the study.

While initial weight loss on a low-calorie diet such as a 1,200-calorie diet is typically rapid and significant, studies have shown that it is typically followed by greater weight gain, some of which is associated with diets that involve only minimal calorie restriction.

In a second study involving 57 overweight or obese individuals, researchers discovered that, on average, participants regained 50 percent of the weight they lost within 10 months.

This explains why low-calorie diets promote metabolic changes that store energy and inhibit weight loss. These changes include an increase in hunger, a loss of lean body mass, and a reduction in the number of actual calories burned, all of which make it more difficult to maintain a healthy weight over time.

Consequently, many health professionals now recommend eating patterns that employ a modest reduction in caloric intake to promote weight loss while minimizing the detrimental metabolic adaptations associated with low-calorie diets. These eating practices have been found to aid in weight loss.

Accelerates Weight Loss

The only way to lose weight effectively and permanently is to expend more calories per day than you consume. This can be accomplished by either increasing your regular physical activity or decreasing your caloric intake. The majority of individuals can attain a caloric deficit, which may aid in weight loss, by consuming only 1,200 calories per day. According to the findings of a Montreal-based study, adhering to a low-calorie diet for a brief period will help reduce abdominal obesity and result in an average of 8% weight loss. Following a nutrient-dense 1,200-calorie diet could result in a weekly weight loss of one to two pounds, depending on your metabolism and nutritional requirements. T

CHAPTER 3: CAN IT AID IN WEIGHT LOSS?

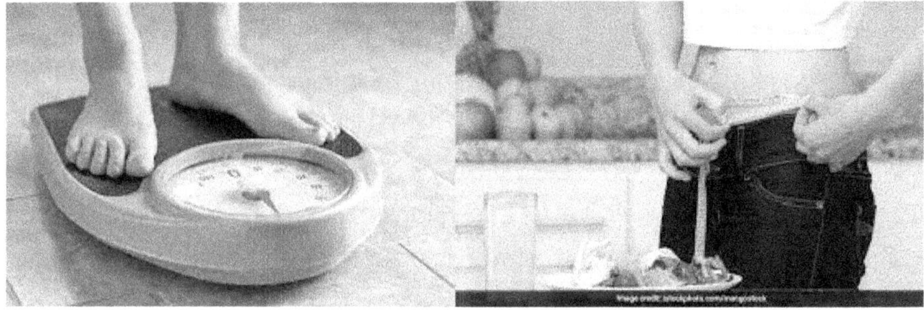

The creation of a calorie deficit is required for successful weight loss. Some medical professionals assert that reducing daily caloric intake by 500 to 750 calories is the most effective strategy for short-term weight loss. In a separate study, adults were assigned one of three weight-loss regimens: 500 calories per day, 1,200–1,500 calories per day, or 1,500–1,800 calories per day. Those who adhered to a 1,200– 1,500-calorie-per-day diet for one year lost an average of 15 pounds (6.8 kg). In contrast, 23 percent of the 4,588 participants who were consuming a 1,200-calorie diet bowed out of the study.

While initial weight loss on a low-calorie diet such as a 1,200-calorie diet is typically rapid and significant, studies have shown that it is typically followed by greater weight gain, some of which is associated with diets that involve only minimal calorie restriction.

In a second study involving 57 overweight or obese individuals, researchers discovered that, on average, participants regained 50 percent of the weight they lost within 10 months.

This explains why low-calorie diets promote metabolic changes that store energy and inhibit weight loss. These changes include an increase in hunger, a loss of lean body mass, and a reduction in the number of actual calories burned, all of which make it more difficult to maintain a healthy weight over time.

As a result, many health professionals now propose eating patterns that employ just a slight decrease in calorie intake to facilitate weight loss while reducing the detrimental metabolic adaptations associated with low-calorie diets. These eating practices have been found to aid in weight loss. Accelerates Weight Loss

The only way to lose weight effectively and permanently is to expend more calories per day than you consume. This can be accomplished by either increasing your regular physical activity or decreasing your caloric intake. The majority of individuals can attain a caloric deficit, which may aid in weight loss, by consuming only 1,200 calories per day. According to the findings of a Montreal-based study, adhering to a low-calorie diet for a brief period will help reduce abdominal obesity and result in an average of 8% weight loss. Following a nutrient-dense 1,200-calorie diet could result in a weekly weight loss of one to two pounds, depending on your metabolism and nutritional requirements.

CHAPTER 4: RECIPES FOR BREAKFAST

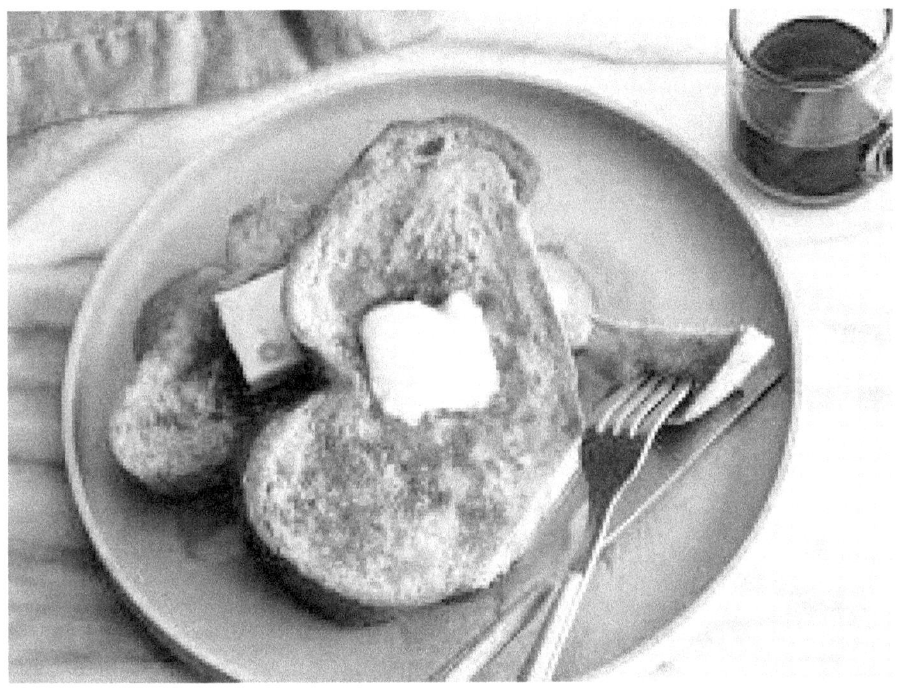

Baked beans

These beans, which don't include any meat, are rich in protein and fiber. If you're seeking a filling vegetarian dish, you've found it.

Servings: Eight

Time Spent Preparing: 30 minutes

Time Spent Cooking: 4 hours 20 minutes

Ingredients:

dry pinto beans, 3/4 cup

Dry red kidney beans, 3/4 cup

dried navy beans, 3/4 cup

5 cups of vegetable stock low in salt

one medium onion peeled and cut in half. one-third cup of molasses

1/fourth cup of Dijon mustard a pinch of salt

1/2 cup of diced tomatoes from cans Apple cider vinegar, 1 tbsp

Directions:

After selecting and sorting beans, soak them overnight.

Set the oven to 250°F.

Beans should be drained and added to a big saucepan with vegetable stock. The mixture should be brought to a boil over high heat and simmered for 30 minutes.

Drain and keep stock in reserve.

In a 2 12 quart baking dish, add beans and onion.

the remaining ingredients together. Pour over the beans, completely encasing them. Cover the pan and bake for 4 hours, checking every half hour to see if more saved stock is necessary.

Nutritional details:

250 calories Fat: 1g

13g of protein

49g of carbohydrates

Stroganoff with beef and spinach

I ate a lot of beef stroganoff over egg noodles when I was younger.

Simply by leaving out the flour that is typically added to thicken the sauce, this dish became low-carb. You won't even be thinking about the egg noodles if you serve this over mashed cauliflower or cabbage noodles.

Serving Size: 2; 10 minutes are required for preparation. 10 minutes for cooking

Ingredients:

8 ounces of sirloin steak, cut into slices that are 12 inches thick.

Sea salt, 1 teaspoon

freshly ground black pepper, one teaspoon

1 tablespoon of extra virgin olive oil or avocado oil

Sliced white mushrooms, 1 cup

12 a finely sliced white onion

2 finely sliced garlic cloves

a quarter cup of low-carb white wine

1/4 cup of sour cream and 1/2 cup of half-and-half smoky paprika, plus an additional for serving 1 teaspoon

Baby spinach, 4 cups

two tablespoons of freshly chopped parsley

Directions:

Salt and pepper should be used to season the steak.

Heat the oil in a medium skillet. When the beef slices have begun to brown, add them and cook for about 5 minutes, rotating them halfway through. Transfer to a plate, then reserve.

Cook the mushrooms, onion, and garlic in the same medium-sized skillet for 5 minutes, or until the onions turn translucent.

After adding the wine, simmer for about two minutes.

Turn down the heat to medium-low and add the steak and any liquids back to the skillet. When the sauce has thickened and the sirloin is fork-tender, add the half-and-half, sour cream, and paprika. Simmer for 8 to 10 minutes.

Place the steak and gravy on top of the spinach in two bowls. Add some parsley and smoked paprika as a garnish.

Nutritional details:
   245 calories Fat: 11g
   39g of protein
   41g of carbohydrates

Mac and cheese baked

This beloved comfort dish is no longer bad for your diet. You don't have to give up on your weight loss objectives to indulge in your love of creamy pasta.

Servings Per Bowl: 4

20 minutes for preparation Preparation Time: 55 minutes

Ingredients:

Two cups of fat-free or reduced-fat ricotta cheese skim milk, divided into 1 12 cups

All-purpose flour, 1 tablespoon

2 cups boiled elbow macaroni

1 1/2 cups of shredded mozzarella or cheddar cheese that is low-fat or fat-free 1 cup of toasty dry breadcrumbs

To taste, add salt and pepper.

Directions:

Ricotta and 1/2 cup milk should be combined in a medium bowl and thoroughly mixed. Flour and 1/4 cup milk should be combined and thoroughly blended in a separate basin.

Then, add the ricotta and flour mixtures and whisk until the remaining milk is smooth and thick. Toss the spaghetti with the milk and cheese mixture.

Bake for 25 minutes after pouring into the baking dish and adding the last of the cheese. Add breadcrumbs and bake for a further five minutes, or until the crumbs are browned. When serving, season with salt and pepper as desired.

Nutritional details:

380 calories Fat: 11g

35g of protein

78g of carbohydrates

Lasagna with aubergine

Want some lasagna? Try this delicious, substantial low-fat dish to avoid the fat and calories you don't want. By substituting aubergine for pasta strands, you may reduce calories while still upping fiber and flavor.

Servings: six

20 minutes for preparation

1 hour for cooking

Ingredients:

Slices of one medium aubergine, each 14-inch thick Juice of two teaspoons of lemon frying oil

Tomato sauce, 2 cups

1 can of chopped whole tomatoes

2 minced garlic cloves

Red chili flakes, 1/4 teaspoon

1 teaspoon basil

Oregano, 1 tablespoon

one-third cup of breadcrumbs

14 cups of shredded fat-free Parmesan cheese

1 cup of ricotta cheese without the fat

1 cup of shredded fat-free mozzarella cheese

Directions:

After spraying the baking sheet with cooking spray, set the sliced aubergine on it and brush it with lemon juice. Cook for roughly 10 minutes, rotating after 5 minutes, until tender.

Tomato sauce, diced tomatoes, garlic, chili flakes, oregano, and basil should all be combined in a bowl. Place aside.

In a bowl, mix the Parmesan and breadcrumbs. Place aside. In a bowl, mix ricotta and mozzarella cheese. Place aside.

Spray cooking spray in a 9-inch square pan. Start by layering the sauce mixture, followed by the eggplant pieces, ricotta mixture, and mozzarella mixture. Continue until every ingredient has been utilized.

45 minutes in the oven after spreading the breadcrumb mixture over top.

Nutritional details:

170 calories Fat: 0.5g

14g of protein

24g of carbohydrates

Wonton Ravioli with Ground Pork

Wonton wrappers can be used in place of pasta to create low-fat ravioli that taste just as delicious when filled with a flavorful pork and shrimp mixture.

Servings: six

Time Spent Preparing: 30 minutes 30 minutes for cooking

Ingredients:

8 ounces of pork

ground Shrimp, 4 ounces

1 chopped green onion, fine

2 minced garlic cloves

1 inch of freshly cut, peeled, and minced ginger

one egg white

Cornflour, 1 teaspoon

Garlic-chili paste, 1 teaspoon a quarter of a lemon's juice

Low-sodium soy sauce, 1 tbsp

a dash of black pepper and salt

One tablespoon of dried and crushed shiitake

mushrooms oil from 2 drops of toasted sesame

3 large, finely shredded Savoy cabbage leaves

36 wrappers for round wontons

Directions:

To make a paste, combine all the ingredients in a food processor, excluding the cabbage and wrappers.

Fold in the cabbage shreds.

Put a wonton wrapper on the counter or cutting board. In the center of each wonton, place 1 spoonful of the prepared filling.

Before covering with a second wonton, dab some cold water along the wonton's edges. Remove all air with caution, then close the borders.

Stock or poach in water till they float.

Nutritional details:
130 calories Fat: 3g
5g protein
6g of carbohydrates

Vegetables roasted in herbs

The preparation of roasted aubergine is quick and varied. The secret to this recipe is to cover every square inch of the fleshy side of the aubergine with fresh herbs and olive oil. Eat it by itself or with some cheese and your preferred spaghetti sauce.
Servings Per Bowl: 4
20 minutes for preparation
hour and 10 minutes for cooking

Ingredients:
aubergines Salt
Extra virgin olive oil, 4 tablespoons

4 teaspoons of garlic, chopped

2 teaspoons of freshly chopped rosemary

2 teaspoons of freshly chopped thyme black pepper freshly ground

Directions:

Set the oven to 400°F. Use parchment paper to line a baking sheet.

The eggplants should be split lengthwise. On the cut side of each aubergine half, make deep cuts in the form of a diamond pattern. Salt the aubergine, then let it aside for 30 minutes to allow any extra liquid to drain.

Squeeze the aubergine as much as you can to get rid of the juice.

Sprinkle the prepared olive oil on the cut side of the eggplant slices and season with salt, pepper, rosemary, and garlic, making sure to get the seasonings into the cracks and crevices.

Bake the eggplant halves for 50 to 60 minutes, or until they are soft, by placing them cut-side down on the prepared baking sheet.

Nutritional details:

204 calories Fat: 9.2g

1.1g of protein

15.7g of carbohydrates

Potato pancakes

It's not necessary to drown potato pancakes in oil for them to be crispy. In this recipe, making a great pancake without frying only requires a small bit of butter and a nonstick pan.

Servings Per Bowl: 4

Time Spent Preparing: 10 minutes 15 minutes for cooking

Ingredients:
1/4 of a yellow onion, grated, and 1 large potato, peeled and shredded

1 ounce of egg

replacement Nutmeg pinch

Fifty-two grams of flour

a single spoonful of fat-free Camembert cheese

1 tbsp. dried chives

1 tablespoon melted butter

freshly ground pepper

Directions:
To make a batter, put all the ingredients in a bowl.

Cooking spray a nonstick skillet, then place it over medium heat.

Pour 1/4 cup of batter onto the pan, cook for around minutes or until golden brown, flip, and cook for another 4 minutes or so.

Serve with low-fat sour cream and applesauce.

Nutritional details:
190 calories Fat: 3.5g 3g. protein

12g of carbohydrates

White bean salad with seared tuna

You enjoy tuna but are sick of tuna salad. For a novel way to eat this fish that is suitable for a diet, try this seared tuna.

Serving Size: 2; 30-minute preparation time 1 hour for cooking

2 fresh (4-ounce) ahi tuna steaks are the ingredients. 1 spoonful of ready pesto with basil

Canola oil, 1 teaspoon

To taste, add salt and pepper.

Julienned and seeded half a red bell pepper

12 green bell pepper, seeded, and thinly julienned; 14 red onion 1/4 cup of grated carrots

Olives from Kalamata, 1/4 cup

12 cups sliced and seeded plum tomatoes

12 cups of prepared balsamic vinegar reduced-fat 12 cups of torn fresh basil leaves

Directions:

Rub pesto all over the tuna, then let it set for an hour.

For a medium rare, season the tuna with salt and pepper before adding it to the hot oil and cooking for 1 1/2 to 2 minutes per side. Take out of the pan and set on a plate.

Then add basil and pour over the tuna. Combine all remaining ingredients (apart from basil) and throw in a heated pan for 30-45 seconds to heat through.

Nutritional details:

390 calories, 15g of fat 36g of protein

25g of carbohydrates

Clams and mussels in a tomato and olive sauce

This recipe is quick and simple to make, yet it tastes like it took hours to make.
Servings Per Bowl: 4

Time Spent Preparing: 10 minutes 20 minutes for cooking

Ingredients:
   2 tablespoons of canola oil,
   34 pounds of fresh mussels,
   34 pounds of fresh clams
   3 crushed garlic cloves with 1/4 cup white wine
   Lemon juice, 1 tablespoon
   12 cups pitted black olives
   1 cup of chopped fresh plum tomatoes
   one cup of low-sodium seafood or vegetable stock
   1 lemon's zest
   Red chili flakes, 1/8 teaspoon
   5 teaspoons chopped fresh parsley

Directions:
   Clams and mussels can be cleaned by soaking them in cold running water.
Throw away any cracked or open shells.

Garlic and chili flakes are added to the heated oil in the preheated sauté pan.
Shellfish must steam for 5 to 8 minutes before they open.
   Serve in a bowl with parsley and crusty bread.

Nutritional details:
   250 calories Fat: 12g
   23g of protein
   10 mg of carbohydrates

Cod Poached in Tomato-Basil

This light fish is given flavor by the addition of hot garlic, sweet tomatoes, and aromatic basil. Serve with the remaining white wine from the bottle, Mediterranean Zucchini Hummus, and various raw vegetables for a cool summer dinner.

Servings Per Bowl: 4

Time Spent Preparing: 10 minutes

Time Spent Cooking: 4 hours 20 minutes

Ingredients:
   Extra virgin olive oil, 1/4 cup
   1 tablespoon of garlic mince
   Half a pound of grape tomatoes a quarter cup of dry white wine
   One lemon's juice and zest
   1 cup of freshly minced basil
   4 fish fillets, 6 ounces each
   table salt
   black pepper freshly ground

Directions:
   Heat the pan with oil. Cook the tomatoes and garlic together until the tomatoes are tender. Wine, white, is added. 2 minutes of simmering is required to cook off some of the alcohol. Flip, then continue cooking until a fork can easily flake the cod.

Nutritional details:
   252 calories Fat: 4g
   27.8g of protein

31g of carbohydrates

CHAPTER 5: RECIPES FOR LUNCH

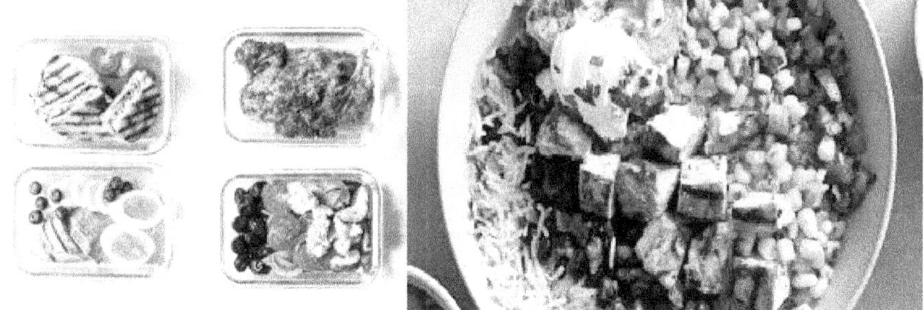

Edamame and Soba with Asian flank steak

The sesame, teriyaki, and chili paste in this meal will appeal to those who like Asian flavors. Servings Per Bowl: 4

Time Spent Preparing: 10 minutes

30 minutes for cooking
   Ingredients:
   Soba noodles weighing 14 pound

Canola oil, 1 teaspoon

a 4-ounce trimmed beef flank steak, thinly sliced against the grain.

Lime juice, 1 1/2 tablespoons

Low-sodium teriyaki sauce, 1 1/2 teaspoons

1 1/2 tablespoons of chili paste and garlic

Cornflour, half a teaspoon

Sesame oil, 1/2 teaspoon 1

2 julienned red pepper

8 strips of snow peas,

2 green onions cut diagonally

1/4 cup of grated carrots

1 cup of thawed frozen edamame

fresh ginger root, chopped, in one spoonful

1/4 cup cilantro

Directions:

Follow the instructions on the soba noodle packet for preparation.

Warm up an oil-filled sauté pan while the noodles are cooking. Cook steak in a pan for about two minutes, or until it's barely done.

To make a sauce, combine lime juice, teriyaki, chili paste, ginger root, cornflour, and sesame oil.

Add the prepared sauce to the pan along with the red pepper, onions, snow peas, and carrot. 2 minutes to cook.

Recycle the beef and plate juices in the pan. Edamame is added and heated thoroughly. Noodles and soba are added; toss. Serve with fresh cilantro as a garnish.

Nutritional details:

31g of carbohydrates

230 calories; 17g protein Fat: 4g

Vegetables that are baked simple and nutritious

Servings: Eight

5 minutes for preparation Preparation Time: 25 minutes

Ingredients:
1 wedged onion, sliced
4 sliced potatoes and 6 sliced carrots
6 cubed chicken breast fillets, cut
Thyme, 1 teaspoon
12 cup water

Directions:
Set the oven to 400 °F.

Put potatoes, carrots, and onion in a baking dish. On top, arrange the chicken.

Thyme, pepper, and water are combined in a basin; add to the chicken; and bake for an hour. Place in a food container and store in the fridge for up to two days.

Before serving, reheat.

Nutritional details: 240 calories
13 mg. cholesterol 25g of carbohydrates Fat: 3.5g

Recipe Buffalo wings

Buffalo wings don't need to be oily and deep-fried to be good. Servings Per Bowl: 4

20 minutes for preparation 50 minutes for cooking

Ingredients:

12 giant chicken wings with the skin off

Black peppercorns, 1 tablespoon

1 small onion

a single celery stalk

1 half head of garlic

2 batch of Spicy and Hot Marinade

2 tablespoons of spicy rub or creole seasoning

Directions: Cook chicken wings for 12 minutes in a heavy, deep saucepan with peppercorns, onions, celery, and garlic.

Cool chicken after removing it from the water.

Let the meat marinate in the hot and spicy marinade over the night. Set the oven to 350°F.

Lay wings in a single layer on a sheet pan, season with Creole seasoning, and bake for 12 minutes. Spray pan with nonstick spray. Serve with the low-fat blue cheese dressing and prepared celery sticks.

Information on nutrition: 230 calories Fat: 5g

21g of protein

12g of carbohydrates

Rice with Curried Chicken Meatballs

These chicken meatballs are a fantastic treat if you like curry. These meatballs contain the flavor you want and the protein you want.

Servings Per Bowl: 4

Time Spent Preparing: 10 minutes 20 minutes for cooking

Ingredients:
   pound of lean chicken ground
   12 cups minced yellow onions
   1/4 cup chopped cilantro
   three tablespoons of plain low-fat yogurt
   1/4 teaspoon of cumin and three tablespoons of flour
   1/4 tsp. of turmeric
   1/4 teaspoon of garam masala and 1/4 teaspoon of ground coriander
   1 tiny serrano chili, chopped after being seeded
   minced garlic cloves
   1/4 cup of egg-free milk

Instructions:
   Combine all ingredients and thoroughly stir.

Bake the meatballs for 7 minutes on a sheet pan that has been sprayed. Put the curry sauce in a saucepan and heat it to a simmer.
   Put cooked meatballs over rice and top with curry sauce.

Nutritional details:
   210 calories Fat: 10g
   22g of protein
   9g of carbohydrates

A casserole with green beans

This beloved family dish doesn't require fried onions to be delicious.

Without frying, the breadcrumbs and raw onions in this dish add wonderful flavor. 8 servings; 15 minutes to prepare.

Preparation Time: 25 minutes

Ingredients:

1/2 yellow onion

thinly sliced Butter,

two tablespoons breadcrumbs, 1 cup

12 cups of fat-free Camembert cheese

1 cup of cream of mushroom soup that is low in fat or fat-free

1/2 cup skim milk

a smidge of soy sauce freshly ground pepper

4 cups of frozen and thawed green beans

sliced one teaspoon of dried thyme

Directions:

Breadcrumbs and Parmesan are added after sautéing onions in butter.

Bake for 20 to 25 minutes, then sprinkle breadcrumbs and onion mixture on top.

Nutritional details:

350 calories Fat: 6g

6g protein

20g of carbohydrates

Chicken Breasts With A Nut Crust

It resembles fried chicken in flavor, but it is low in fat and doesn't involve frying.

Servings Per Bowl: 4

Time Spent Preparing: 25 minutes 20 minutes for cooking

Ingredients:
2 chicken breasts, both skinless and boneless, lightly pounded to an even thickness
1/4 cup flour
Three ounces of liquid egg substitute
To taste, add salt and pepper.
1/4 tsp. of cinnamon
1/4 tsp. of dried thyme
Dry mustard, 1/4 teaspoon
Cayenne pepper, 1/8 teaspoon
12 cups of pecans, walnuts, almonds, or pistachios that have been extremely finely chopped
Canola oil, 2 tablespoons
Maple syrup, 4 tablespoons
1/fourth cup of Dijon mustard

Directions:
Chicken should be lightly dusted in flour and then coated in a beaten egg substitute.

Add the chopped nuts to a medium bowl along with the salt, pepper, cinnamon, thyme, dry mustard, and cayenne.

Cover the chicken entirely with the nut mixture by dredging (dipping) it there. Oil should be heated in a nonstick pan over medium heat.

Place the chicken in the pan and heat for 2–3 minutes, or until the nuts are browned, then turn it over and cook for an additional 2–3 minutes. Finally, bake the chicken for 5-7 minutes.

For the final two minutes of baking, pour over the chicken.

Nutritional details:
   320 calories
   Fat: 16g
   20g of protein 2g of fiber

Roast Pork Loin with Garlic and Rosemary

While being healthful enough to regularly appear on your dinner table, this pork loin is delectable enough to offer at a dinner party.

Servings: Eight

Time Spent Preparing: 22 minutes Preparation Time: 45 minutes

Ingredients:
   chopped rosemary, 3 teaspoons
   4 minced garlic cloves
   split into two teaspoons of kosher salt
   Black pepper, half a teaspoon
   1 (2-pound) center-cut, boneless pork loin roast with visible fat removed
divided into 4 teaspoons of extra virgin olive oil

Directions:

Combine the rosemary, garlic, salt, and pepper in a small bowl.

30 minutes in the oven after mixing the pork with the rosemary mixture on the meat. Serve.

Nutritional details:
    290 calories Fat: 18g
    30g of protein
    1g of carbohydrates

Chicken Braised in Rosemary with Mushroom Sauce

Dieters everywhere should be on the lookout for anything with the word "sauce" in it. Typically, sauces are either fatty, salty or have enough calories to constitute a meal on their own.

Servings Per Bowl: 4

Timing for Preparation: 15 minutes 30 minutes for cooking

Ingredients:
    Boneless, skinless chicken thighs weighing one pound
    Canola oil, 2 tablespoons
    2 pieces of turkey prosciutto or bacon
    1 tiny shallot, chopped, and 1/4 cup of diced yellow onion
    1 smashed garlic clove
    3 fresh rosemary sprigs
    3 ounces of quartered fresh cremini mushrooms
    1 sliced and halved portobello mushroom cap
    Flour, one teaspoon
    1 cup of vegetable stock low in salt

Red wine, half a cup

To taste, add salt and pepper.

Directions:

Chicken should be lightly oiled before being placed in a deep skillet over medium heat to brown all sides (about 5 minutes per side).

For 10 minutes, sauté the bacon with the shallots, onions, garlic, rosemary, and mushrooms.

Add flour, stock, and red wine; cover and simmer for about 10 minutes, or until the liquid is thick and the chicken is done.

Nutritional details:

380 calories

Fat: 21g

33g of protein

9g of carbohydrates

Recipe Steak fajitas

There is no additional fat in this recipe, yet the steak is incredibly juicy.

Servings: Eight

5 minutes for preparation Preparation Time: 25 minutes

Ingredients:

a single onion, sliced

Cut one green bell into strips.

1/2 tsp. of thyme

1/2 tsp. mustard powder

Black pepper, 1 teaspoon

Cumin, 1 teaspoon

2 teaspoons of dried rosemary

Chilli powder, 2 tablespoons

The natural sweetener in two packets Paprika, 1 tablespoon

1/fourth cup of sea salt

Lean sirloin steak weighing 1 pound, sliced into strips

Directions:

To combine, combine the salt, paprika, sweetener, chili powder, dried rosemary, cumin, pepper, mustard powder, and dried thyme in a bowl.

Take one tablespoon of this mixture and set it aside. Heat a big skillet on the hob to a medium-high setting.

Add the spice mixture that you previously left aside to the skillet along with the prepared onion and pepper. The onion and peppers must be cooked until the peppers are tender and the onions are transparent.

Remove from heat and put in a bowl. To remain warm, cover.

Half the seasoned steak should be added to the same skillet and cooked for two minutes on each side, or until done to your preference. Place the finished steak on a clean platter and cover it while the remaining steak cooks.

Add everything back into the skillet and reheat for a few minutes once all the steak strips have been cooked. Put some on plates and eat.

Nutritional details:

401 calories Fat: 22.1g 104.7% protein

6g of carbohydrates

Recipe Tuna Noodle Casserole

Want comfort food but want to stay away from the extra calories and fat? Try this variation on a classic.

Servings: six

20 minutes for preparation Preparation Time: 40 minutes

Ingredients:
   dried wide whole wheat egg noodles,
   6 ounces Canola oil, two teaspoons
   12 cups of softened, finely diced, unpackaged sun-dried tomatoes
   1 small onion, tiny dice
   one red bell pepper, tiny chopped
   1 minced garlic clove
   1 celery stalk, chopped
   two teaspoons of regular flour
   Skim milk in two glasses
   fat-free mayonnaise in a half-cup
   can of spring water, packed with drained tuna (or chicken in a can).
   12 cups of low-fat Swiss cheese, grated
   teaspoons of freshly chopped basil
   Lemon juice, 1 tablespoon
   To taste, add salt and pepper.
   toasted almonds in a third of a cup

Directions:
   The oven should be preheated to 425°F.

Pasta should be cooked for about 6 minutes before draining, rinsing, and setting aside.

Add oil and garlic to a hot pan. After 3 minutes of cooking the vegetables and tomatoes, add the milk and flour and cook for another 4 minutes.

Add the basil, cheese, mayo, and tuna.

Add salt, pepper, and lemon juice for seasoning.

Add almonds, then bake for 20 minutes. 5 minutes should pass before serving.

Nutritional details:
  310 calories Fat: 9g
  23g of protein
  37g of carbohydrates

CHAPTER 6: RECIPES FOR DINNER

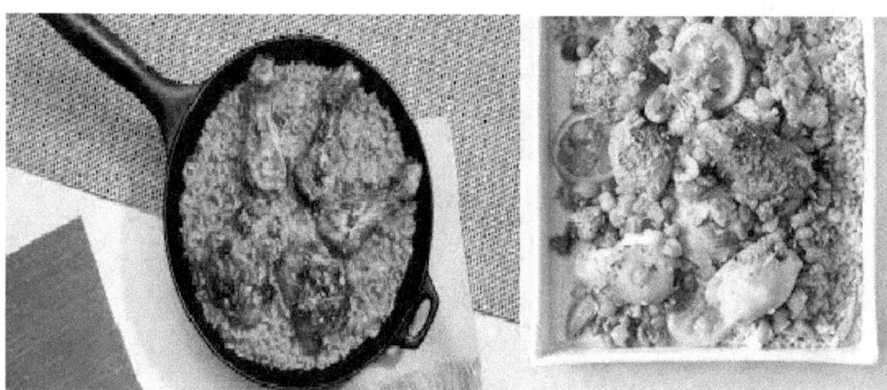

African Chicken and Rice

Recipes for low-fat chicken frequently come out dry and flavourless. Chillis, tomatoes, and chicken stock are used in this dish to boost flavour and keep the chicken moist in order to make up for the flavour lost to fat.

Servings: six

20 minutes for preparation 35 minutes for cooking
Ingredients:
1/4 tsp. dry thyme

1 cooked cup of white rice

Low-sodium chicken stock, 1 quart

Tomato paste, 2 tablespoons

1 smashed garlic clove

cup of diced tomato from a can Vegetable oil

1 tablespoon diced one medium onion

tablespoons of dried prawns, ground

12 of a chopped and seeded serrano pepper

Boneless, skinless chicken breast weighing 2 pounds

Directions:

Heat the pan with oil

Thyme and garlic should be combined, then applied to the chicken.

Chicken should be cooked for three minutes on each side in hot oil with onion, tomato paste, and diced tomato.

After that, add the stock, chilli and dried prawns, and simmer for 15 minutes. Add chicken and sauce to the rice before serving.

Nutritional details:

410 calories Fat: 8g

51g of protein

32g of carbohydrates

Chicken and vegetables Unfried Rice

Do you crave fried rice but are aware that anything with the term "fried" in the title can't be good for your diet? Try this low-fat recipe for fried rice to get all the flavour and none of the calories or fat found in restaurants.

Servings Per Bowl: 4

20 minutes for preparation 20 minutes for cooking

Ingredients:
  Three ounces of liquid egg substitute
  2 chicken breasts, thinly sliced
  1 minced garlic clove
  Garlic-chili paste, 1/4 teaspoon
  12 cup of thawed frozen mixed vegetables
  1/2 yellow onion, chopped finely
  fresh bean sprouts, 1/4 cup
  Low-sodium soy sauce, 1 tbsp
  Sesame oil, 1/2 teaspoon
  2 cups of chilled, cooked brown rice

Directions:
  Apply cooking spray to a nonstick pan, add the liquid eggs, and cook over low heat until a single sheet of cooked egg forms (much like an omelette). If necessary, finish in the oven.

Take out the eggs, let them cool, then flip them over and cut them into strips.

the pan with oil, add the chicken, garlic, and chilli paste, and cook for three minutes. For an additional 2 minutes, add the onion, frozen veggies, and bean sprouts.
  After heating the rice, soy sauce, and sesame oil, add the egg strips last and stir to incorporate. Serve warm.

Nutritional details:
  27g of carbohydrates Fat: 3g
  19g of protein 220 calories

Alfredo sauce over pasta

This sauce is a low-fat adaptation of a traditionally high-fat pasta meal.
Servings: two

Timing for Preparation: 15 minutes Preparation Time: 25 minutes

Ingredients:

Cooking oil substitute

2 minced garlic cloves

Cream cheese without fat, two tablespoons

1 and a third cups of skim milk

two teaspoons of regular flour

2 tablespoons of butter (or butter replacement) sprinkling 1 cup of low-fat or fat-free food Camembert cheese

black pepper, to taste

2 cups of any type of cooked pasta

Directions:

Apply cooking spray to a nonstick skillet. Cook the garlic until it is soft on a low heat setting. Over medium heat, stir in the milk, cream cheese, and flour before bringing to a boil.

Stir in the Parmesan cheese, black pepper, and butter sprinklings. Add right away and coat pasta with.

Nutritional details:

440 calories Fat: 1.5g

27g of protein

60g of carbohydrates

Roasted pork shoulder

This serving size is adequate for a modest dinner gathering. After cooking, the roast will reduce by about half, leaving two to three pounds of tasty but affordable pork roast.

Servings Per Bowl: 12

18 minutes for preparation 35 minutes for cooking

Ingredients:
   10 minced garlic cloves
   2 teaspoons of fresh rosemary
   2 tablespoons of freshly chopped sage
   1 tablespoon of roasted fennel seeds
   Kosher salt, 1 1/2 teaspoons
   1/14th cup of black pepper
   1/4 cup of orange juice
   2 cups of cider apple
   1 4- to 5-pound pork shoulder roast tied by the butcher
   3 Granny Smith apples, cored and cut in half

Directions:
   In a food processor, combine the sage, rosemary, garlic, fennel, salt, pepper, orange juice, and apple cider; process until a paste forms. Pork roast should be covered in paste.

Place the apples in the roasting pan and place the roast on top.

On the middle rack of the oven, cover and bake for six hours. Take meat out of oven when internal temperature reaches 175°F and it can be easily torn with a fork. Let it rest for 15 minutes.

With a fork, shred the meat and serve.

Nutritional details:
310 calories Fat: 12g
38g of protein
11g of carbohydrates

Pork Tenderloin with Cherry Sauce

Pork tenderloin is a fantastic family dish because it is the ideal size to serve four people. Additionally being a particularly lean pork cut, tenderloin is a fantastic option for your diet.

Servings Per Bowl: 4

Time Spent Preparing: 10 minutes 28 minutes for cooking

Ingredients:
Pork tenderloin, not pork loin, 1 pound
1/4 teaspoon salt
freshly ground black pepper, 1/4 teaspoon
2 shallots, sliced
Olive oil, 1 teaspoon
Dried cherries, half a cup
Low-sodium chicken stock, 1 cup
Balsamic vinegar, 3 tablespoons
tarragon, 1 teaspoon
pomegranate juice, 1/4 cup

Directions:
In a big sauté pan, lightly season the prepared pork with salt and pepper

before searing. For 2 minutes, sauté cherries in oiled pan.

Bring to a boil after adding the last of the prepared ingredients. Sliced pork should be topped with sauce.   48

Nutritional details: 32g of carbohydrates 26g of protein
   Fat: 6g
   280 calories

CHAPTER 7: SOUP RECIPES

Cheesy Cauliflower Soup

Even though he dislikes veggies, my father usually requests more of this soup. 8 servings; 20 minutes for preparation.

Preparation Time: 45 minutes

Ingredients:
   Olive oil, 3 tablespoons
   1/4 cup finely chopped onions
   Five cups of chicken
   stock water, 1 cup
   florets from 1 medium cauliflower
   rosemary, 1/8 teaspoon
   2 cups of shredded cheddar cheese
   1/8 teaspoon thyme
   Black pepper, 1/4 teaspoon
   Melted 2 tablespoons of butter
   14 cups of whole wheat flour

Directions:

Onions should be cooked for around five minutes over medium heat once the pan has been oiled and heated.

Cauliflower, water, rosemary, thyme, and pepper should all be added. Cook the cauliflower, covered, for about 30 minutes on low heat, or until soft. Get rid of the heat.

Return the mixture to the heat after mashing the cauliflower with a potato masher until it is broken up into small bits.

Melted butter and flour should be combined in a small bowl and thoroughly mixed before being added to the soup. The soup should be thickened to the appropriate consistency by stirring constantly over low heat.

One cup of cheese at a time, add while stirring until melted. Serve.

Nutritional details:
252 calories, 14g of total fat, 24g of total carbohydrate, and 0g of protein.

Soup with Chicken and Beans

For me, it was love at first bite with this soup. Because conventional bacon softens in soup, I typically substitute vegan bacon in its stead.

servings per recipe: 4; 15 minutes for preparation. Preparation Time: 40 minutes

Ingredients:
One tablespoon of olive oil
1/2 cup finely chopped onion
a single minced garlic clove

1 can of flavor-infused chicken broth with roasted vegetables and herbs

12 cup water

1 cup of washed and drained canned great northern beans cooked and finely chopped 1/4 cup of chicken

Black pepper, 1/4 teaspoon

1 strip of cooked and finely crushed vegetarian bacon

Directions:

Heat oil in a medium saucepan; add onion and garlic; cook over low heat for 5 minutes or until tender. In a pan, boil water and broth.

Cook for 30 minutes after adding the last few ingredients. sometimes stir.

Nutritional details:

Total Fat: 5.7g, Carbohydrate: 39g, Protein: 4.6g, Calories: 225.7 Recipe Chicken-

Barley Soup

A filling soup that makes you feel fulfilled. To ensure that the barley is perfectly soft, let this soup simmer for a few hours. The barley will continue to soften throughout the night, making this soup even creamier the next day.

Servings: Eight

20 minutes for preparation

Cooking time: one hour

Ingredients:

one pound of chicken ground

1 cup of a vegetable juice mixture, such as V8, two (14-ounce) cans of chicken broth 4 cups of liquid

1 cup of finely sliced, peeled, and chopped carrots

12 cups of finely shredded cabbage

12 cups chopped green pepper

1 cup of finely chopped onion

2 minced garlic cloves

seasoned salt, two teaspoons

uncooked barley, 3/4 cup

Directions:

In a sizable saucepan over medium heat, cook the prepared ground chicken, turning frequently, until the chicken is browned and crumbly. Remove fat.

As you add the broth, juice, water, carrots, cabbage, green pepper, onion, and garlic, stir in the barley. Use seasoned salt to season. Cover the pot and boil the barley for 1 to 2 hours over low heat, stirring occasionally.

Nutritional details:

90 calories worth of total fat, 3 grams worth of carbs. 10.5 g Protein

Chicken Noodle Soup

Using home-cooked chicken and homemade broth will give this soup a richer flavor. Even one cup of homemade stock, along with one cup of canned broth, will help give this delightful "comfort" soup a homemade flavor.

Servings: Eight

Time Spent Preparing: 30 minutes

Time Spent Cooking: 1 Hour 30 Minutes

Ingredients:
   one tablespoon of canola or olive oil
   1/4 cup finely chopped onion
   2/3 cup of shredded carrots four cups of chicken stock
   2 glasses of water
   1 tablespoon of flakes of dried celery
   Bay leaf, one
   1 cup of chopped, cooked chicken
   1 tablespoon of flakes of parsley
   14 teaspoons of black pepper, or to taste
   1 teaspoon of seasoned salt Uncooked
   broken egg
   noodles, 1 1/2 cups, in 3-inch pieces.

Directions:

Oil, carrots, and onion should all be added to a big saucepan and cooked for 5 minutes.

Add the chicken, water, bay leaf, celery flakes, and broth. Cook for an hour while stirring occasionally.

Noodles, parsley, salt, and pepper should all be added at this point. Cook for another 25 minutes on low heat with the lid on. To serve, remove the bay leaf.

Nutritional details:

220 calories, 5g of total fat, 24g of total carbohydrate, and 18g of protein.

Cream of Broccoli Soup

This soup is perfect if you love broccoli. Smoothly blended, it is tasty, easy to consume, and pairs well with your preferred sandwich.

Servings: six

Timing for Preparation: 15 minutes Preparation Time: 45 minutes

Ingredients:
   4 cups of florets from broccoli
   1 cup of chopped onion
   1 tablespoon of flakes from celery
   one sliced garlic clove, and one diced medium potato
   1 chicken broth (14 ounces)
   2glasses of milk
   1 1/2 cups of shredded cheddar cheese
   1/4 tsp. of thyme
   1/4 teaspoon of white pepper and 1/2 teaspoon of salt

Directions:
   In a medium saucepan, combine the broccoli, onion, celery flakes, garlic, potato, and chicken broth. Bring to a boil; then reduce heat, cover, and simmer for 30 minutes.

After the vegetables have been pureed, add the milk, cheese, thyme, salt, and pepper to the pot with the vegetables.

Continue to cook the cheese over a low fire, frequently turning it, until it melts.

Nutritional details:
   168 calories, 7g of total fat, 15g of total carbohydrate, and 5g of protein.

Cream of Potato Soup

This incredibly adaptable recipe is simple to modify to suit your preferences. It can be consumed as a straightforward potato soup or with the addition of gammon, cheese, or veggies. Simply puree or softly mash it in a blender for a smoother soup.

Servings: six

Timing for Preparation: 15 minutes Preparation Time: 45 minutes

Ingredients:
   10 grams of butter
   1 cup of finely chopped onion
   3 cups of potato dice
   1 cup of shredded sharp cheddar cheese (optional)
   14 teaspoons of black pepper and three cups of chicken broth
   1/2 tsp. of salt
   Garlic powder, 1/2 teaspoon
   14 cups whole wheat flour
   1 1/2 cups milk

Directions:
   Butter is heated in a pan. The prepared onion should be added, stirred, and cooked until softened.

Add potatoes, chicken stock, pepper, salt, and garlic powder, along with any more gammon that you desire.

For about 40 minutes, boil the potatoes covered over low heat until they are soft and easily crumble. If desired, add cheese; mix just until melted and smooth. Serve.

Nutritional details:

Total Fat: 5.7g, Carbohydrate: 39g, Protein: 4.6g, Calories: 225.7 Recipe Creamy Chicken

Vegetable Soup

I was taught this recipe by a dental assistant who frequently prepared it for her in-laws when they started to crave soft meals. Both of them and you will enjoy it!

Servings: six

20 minutes for preparation

Time Spent Cooking: 1 Hour 45 Minutes
Ingredients:
Olive oil, 2 tablespoons
1/2 cup finely chopped onions
12 cups of shredded or finely sliced carrots
12 cups diced potatoes
Green beans, 1/2 cup
Peas, half a cup
1 cup of chopped-up chicken
chicken broth in a single (14-ounce) can with a dash of black pepper
1 1/4 cups milk
1 can of cream of celery soup (1034 ounces)
1 can of cream of cheddar cheese soup (1034 ounces)

Instructions:
Heat oil in a big pot; add onions and carrots; and simmer for 5 minutes. Add

the chicken, broth, pepper, potatoes, green beans, and peas. For 112 hours, or until the veggies are tender, cover the pan and cook over low heat while stirring regularly.

Stir in the celery soup, milk, and cheddar cheese soup, and boil until well cooked.

Nutritional details:

128 calories, 3.6g of total fat, 15.6g of total carbohydrate, and 7.6g of protein. Recipe

French Onion Soup

Even though it just contains a few ingredients, French onion soup has a fantastic flavor. For a quick lunch, this soup comes together quite quickly.

Servings: six

Time Spent Preparing: 30 minutes 30 minutes for cooking

Ingredients:
   1/2 cup dry red wine
   four cups of chicken stock
   1 teaspoon of minced, finely ground garlic
   6 1-inch-thick pieces of French bread Olive oil, 1 tbsp
   6 freshly grated teaspoons of parmesan cheese
   2 cups of coarsely chopped sweet onions

Directions:
   Oil and heat the pan with the onions. Include the wine, broth, and garlic. Cook for 25 minutes with the lid on.
   In the meantime, lightly toast the bread, then place a piece in the bottom of

each soup bowl and top with 1 tablespoon of Parmesan cheese.

To serve, ladle soup over toast.

Nutritional details:
190 calories, 9g of total fat, 21g of total carbohydrate, and 7g of protein.

Soup with Ham and Beans

On a chilly day, warming up with this traditional soup is never a mistake. A perfect, straightforward meal can be made by serving cornbread alongside it.

Servings: Eight

Time Spent Preparing: 25 minutes 5 hours for cooking

Ingredients:
(14)-ounce cans of chicken broth and a half (16-ounce) bag of navy beans
2 glasses of water
1 cup of finely sliced carrots
1 cup of finely chopped onion
2 chopped garlic cloves
1 can of chopped tomatoes with juice (14 ounces)
Black pepper, half a teaspoon
seasoned salt, 1 1/2 tablespoons
1 cup of finely chopped green cabbage
5 ounces of smoked ground ham in a can.

Directions:
Navy beans should be washed as directed on the box.

In a pot big enough to handle it, bring one quart of the prepared water to a boil. Add the beans, cover, and remove from the heat after one hour to let the beans soften. Drain them after that.

Add the seasoning packet, along with the ham, cabbage, stock, water, carrots, onion, garlic, tomatoes, pepper, and seasoned salt. For three to four hours, or until the beans are incredibly soft, cook the beans, covered, over low heat. Change things up occasionally.

Nutritional details:

calories 177 total fat grams 2 total carbs 14g Protein, 26g

CHAPTER 8: RECIPE FOR SNACKS

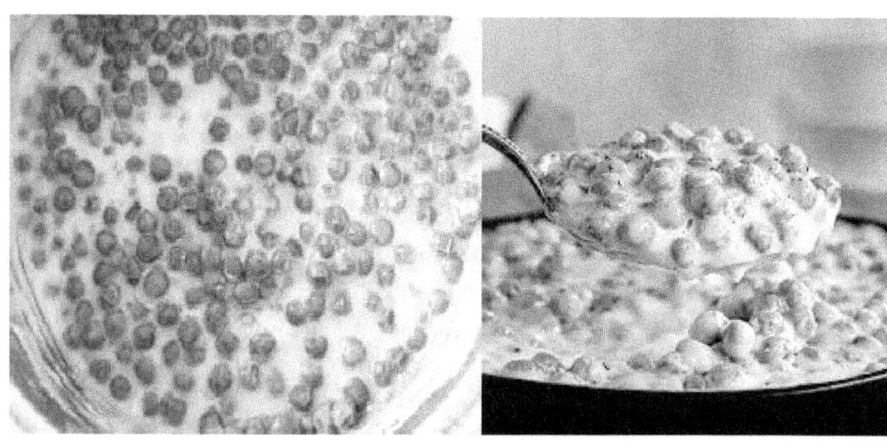

Creamed Peas

Just before serving, purée the dish for an even softer meal.

Servings Per Bowl: 4

Time Spent Preparing: 10 minutes Preparation Time: 25 minutes

Ingredients:

2/3 cup of chicken stock

2 cups of peas, green

Butter, two tablespoons

1/3 cup half-and-half

1/4 teaspoon of black pepper and two tablespoons of flour

1/4 teaspoon salt

Grated Parmesan cheese, 2 teaspoons (optional)

Directions:

Add the stock and peas to a medium saucepan and heat to almost boiling. 25 minutes of cooking at reduced heat.

Half-and-half and flour should be combined in a small bowl before being added to the pea mixture and cooked and stirred until thickened.

Stir in the salt, pepper, and Parmesan cheese, if using, before serving.

Nutritional details:

150 calories

Total Carbohydrates 19g, Total Fat 6.2g, and Protein 5.9g

Creamed Spinach

This is a recipe for creamed spinach that has been around for a long time. 8 servings; 10 minutes for preparation.

10 minutes for cooking

Ingredients:

10 ounce containers of thawed, coarsely chopped

frozen spinach Butter, two tablespoons

1 little clove of garlic, minced

teaspoons of coarsely chopped onion

Sauce:

Butter, two tablespoons

8 grains of nutmeg

Whole flour, two teaspoons

100 ml of milk

1/4 teaspoon salt

Black pepper, 1/8 teaspoon

Directions:

Heat a pan with oil; add the onion and garlic; stir and cook for 5 minutes, or until tender. Add the spinach, mix gently, and transfer to a serving bowl.

In the meantime, melt the butter in a small saucepan over low heat. Add the flour, milk, nutmeg, salt, and pepper. Stir until the mixture reaches the appropriate consistency.

Combine spinach and sauce. Serve.

Nutritional details:

188 calories

Total Carbohydrates 11.94g Protein 6.66g Total Fat 9.02g

Recipe 37. Sandwich with egg salad

A delicious and airy traditional egg salad sandwich. By adding a half-teaspoon of sweet curry powder, you may transform this into curried egg salad. You can also try adding some shredded cheese and boiled peas.

Servings Per Bowl: 4

Timing for Preparation: 15 minutes 1 hour for cooking

Ingredients:
  Mayonnaise, half a cup
  Pickle relish, 2 tablespoons
  Unprepared mustard, 1 teaspoon
  1/4 teaspoon each of salt and black pepper
  8 hard-boiled eggs, sliced and peeled
  1 peeled and thinly sliced tomato Portobello fungi

Directions:
  Mix the mayonnaise, relish, mustard, salt, and pepper in a medium bowl. Gently stir in the diced eggs. To cool, refrigerate.

Place cooled egg salad in portobello mushrooms and, if preferred, top with prepared tomato slices.

Nutritional details:
  220 calories, 9.5g of total fat, 10g of total carbohydrate, and 12.8g of protein.

Cottage cheese with peaches in gelatin

This tasty side dish has been a favourite in our family for years. It is particularly enjoyable on a hot summer day. Before incorporating the cottage cheese and peaches into the gelatin, blend them for an even softer gelatin dessert.

Servings: six

Timing for Preparation: 15 minutes 20 minutes for cooking

Ingredients:

1 (.3-ounce) container of cherry-flavored gelatin is included

1 cup of cottage cheese with tiny curds

1 cup of chopped or sliced peaches

Gelatin should be prepared as directed on the package and chilled in the refrigerator.

Directions:

Slice the peaches into bite-sized pieces while you wait.

Fold in cottage cheese and peaches when the gelatin has almost set. Returned to the refrigerator, firm up.

Nutritional details:

220 calories, 2g of total fat, 16g of total carbohydrate, and 20g of protein.

Sandwich with Ham Salad

This recipe's smoked gammon transforms a straightforward gammon salad into a delectable sandwich. Servings Per Bowl: 4

Timing for Preparation: 15 minutes 30 minutes for cooking

Ingredients:

Five-ounce cans of drained ground smoked ham

2 hard-boiled eggs, cut finely

Mayonnaise, half a cup

Sweet pickle relish, 2 teaspoons

1/2 tsp. of onion powder

Unprepared mustard, 1 teaspoon

Black pepper, 1/4 teaspoon

Shredded half a cup of cheddar cheese is optional

4 grilled, halved portobello mushrooms

Instructions:

In a prepared small basin, whisk together the mayonnaise, pickle relish, onion powder, mustard, and pepper.

Put the mayonnaise mixture over the gammon and eggs and, if you like, the cheese. Mix thoroughly; chill in the refrigerator.

To serve, insert gammon salad inside portobello mushrooms.

Nutritional details:

293 calories, 5g of total carbohydrates, 6.5g of total fat, and 14g of protein.

A piping-hot chicken sandwich

While other hot shredded chicken recipes utilise a can of creamed soup to make a creamier sauce, this family favourite is cooked in broth. Simply reduce the amount of broth and omit the seasoned salt if you'd rather make soup. This sandwich is tasty in either case.

8 servings; 10 minutes for preparation.

15 minutes for cooking

Ingredients:

Finely chopped cooked chicken from 3 1/2 cups or 1 (28-ounce) can of chicken
Chicken broth split into 1 34 cups and crushed half of a sleeve of round buttery crackers a single teaspoon of seasoning salt
Black pepper, 1/4 teaspoon
1 (10 3/4-ounce) low-sodium can of cream of mushroom soup

8 grilled portobello mushrooms, cut in half

Directions:

Chicken, 1 12 cups of broth, cracker crumbs, salt, and pepper are all added to a medium pot and stirred while cooking on low heat.

Add more liquid if it starts to get too dry during cooking. Continue to boil, stirring constantly, until everything is heated through and the chicken is moist and just a little juicy, but not soggy that it soddens the mushrooms.

Serve hot chicken tucked into portobello mushrooms.

Nutritional details:
201 calories
Total Carbohydrates 25.1g Protein 6.5g Total Fat 32.6g

Slices of Marinated Tomato

This dish has a nice appearance and is a straightforward way to appreciate summer's bounty. If you like, serve this with bread or rolls so you can mop up the flavorful sauce.

8 servings; 20 minutes for preparation. 3 hours for cooking

Ingredients:
4 substantial tomatoes
1/4 cup olive oil
Lemon juice, 1 tablespoon
Sugar, 1 teaspoon
1/2 tsp. of salt
1/2 tsp. of oregano 1 teaspoon parsley

Directions:

Layer the tomatoes in an oblong shallow serving dish after peeling and cutting into 1-inch slices.

In a small bowl, combine salt, oregano, lemon juice, oil, sugar, and parsley mix well.

Nutritional details:

58 calories Total Fat 3.7g

Total Carbohydrate 5.9g Protein 0.7g

Potato Salad

A traditional summer side dish, I usually put several hard-boiled eggs in it as my parents sometimes eat a small dish of potato salad as a simple lunch. I use vegetable bacon since it retains its delicious bacon flavour while becoming soft in salad dressing.

Servings: Eight

Time Spent Preparing: 10 minutes 30 minutes for cooking

Ingredients:

Cooked, peeled, and diced 4 medium potatoes

4 hard-boiled eggs, sliced and peeled

Two pieces of crumbled, crisp-cooked vegetable bacon

onion powder, 1 teaspoon

Mayonnaise, half a cup

1/4 cup of Ranch dressing Vinegar

1 1/2 tablespoons Sugar, two tablespoons

Unprepared mustard 1 tbsp

1 teaspoon chives

1 tablespoon grated Parmesan cheese

1/2 tsp. of seasoning salt

Black pepper, 1/4 teaspoon

Directions:

Combine diced potatoes that have cooled, chopped eggs, and crumbled vegetable bacon in a big bowl.

Mayonnaise, Ranch dressing, vinegar, sugar, chives, Parmesan cheese, seasoned salt, and pepper should all be combined in a medium bowl.

Pour the mayonnaise dressing mixture over the potato mixture, gently whisk to blend, then cover and chill.

Nutritional details:

197 calories

11 g of total fat, 18.9 g of total carbohydrate, and 5.8 g of protein

Salad of Soft Cauliflower

A beautiful, soft salad. Servings Per Bowl: 4

20 minutes for preparation 10 minutes for cooking

Ingredients:

3 cups of florets from cauliflower

4 cups of liquid

Bay leaf, one

1/8 teaspoon of thyme or rosemary for the dressing

2 teaspoons of white wine vinegar or balsamic vinegar

Sugar, half a teaspoon

a single minced garlic clove

Black pepper, 1/8 teaspoon

1/2 tsp. of basil

Olive oil, 1/3 cup

1/2 tsp. of oregano

Directions:

Add bay leaf and cauliflower to 4 cups of boiling water.

Remove the bay leaf, cover, and cook the cauliflower over low heat until it is soft. Drain the cauliflower, then put it in a medium bowl and put it in the fridge to cool.

Olive oil, garlic, vinegar, sugar, basil, oregano, thyme, and pepper should all be mixed together in a small bowl.

Pour the dressing over the cauliflower; gently toss to incorporate; then cover and chill in the refrigerator.

Nutritional details:

Total Fat: 6.7g Total Carbohydrate: 14.4g Protein: 4.9g Calories: 125

Brussels sprouts with turkey bacon

The rendered fat from the turkey bacon is used to flavour the often bitter brussel sprouts in these turkey bacon brussel sprouts. Think about adding some apple cider vinegar and crispy turkey bacon bits to the dish to improve the flavour.

Servings Per Bowl: 4

20 minutes for preparation

1 hour and 25 minutes for cooking

Ingredients:

pound of halved and trimmed Brussels sprouts

Butter, two tablespoons

ounces of chopped, fried thick-cut turkey bacon

2 minced garlic cloves

1/4 teaspoon each of salt and pepper

Directions:

Set the water bath's temperature to 183 °F.

All the ingredients should be sealed and submerged in water. Cook for one hour. Set the oven to broil for 5 minutes, or until well cooked. Enjoy!

Nutritional details:

Total Carbohydrate 10.8g, Total Fat 20.2g, and Protein 4g per 230 calories.

CHAPTER 9: MEAL PLANING

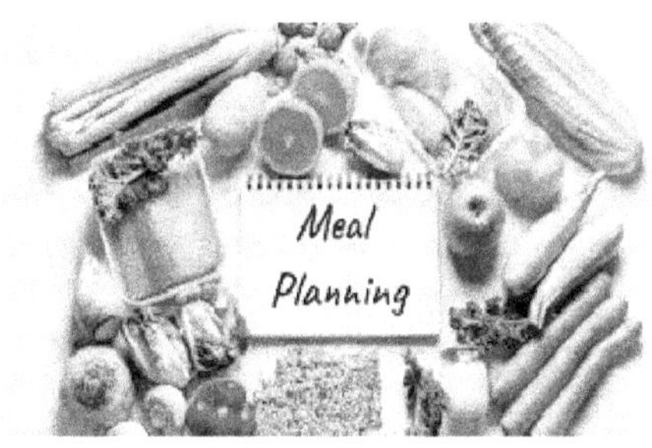
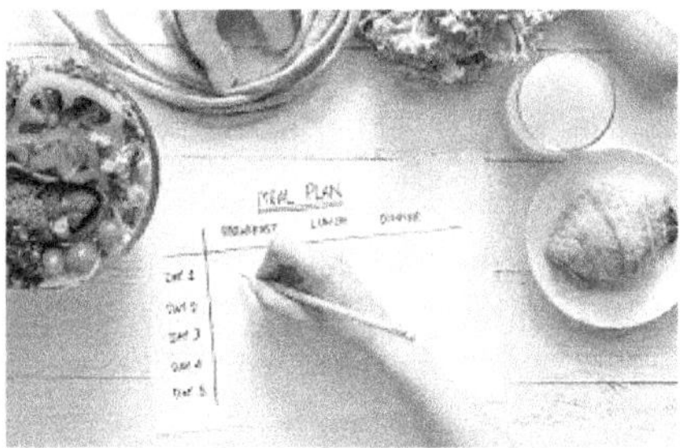

Breakfast: Baked Mac and Cheese (380 calories) from Meal Plan 1.

Buffalo wings for lunch, 230 calories Dinner will be pasta with 440 calories.

Creamed Peas, 150 calories, as a side dish or snack One thousand two hundred calories total.

Meal Plan 2: Tomato-Basil Poached Cod for Breakfast, 252 Calories Lunch: 350-calorie green bean casserole

Dinner: Unfried rice with chicken and vegetables, 220 calories

Sides/Snacks: Hot Shredded Chicken Sandwich with Ham and Bean Soup, 378 calories. One thousand two hundred calories total.

Breakfast on Meal Plan 3: 390 calories of seared tuna and white bean salad Steak Fajitas with 401 calories for lunch

351 calories worth of creamy beef stroganoff with mushrooms for dinner Sides/Snacks: Slices of marinated tomato, 58 calories

One thousand two hundred calories total.

Plan 4 for Meals

250 calories for breakfast: Stewed mussels and clams with tomatoes and olives Lunch: Chicken with mushroom sauce and rosemary braised in 380 calories

Dinner: 260 calorie Chipotle Shredded Pork Sides/Snacks: 310 calorie Chicken Barley Soup + Egg Salad Sandwich

One thousand two hundred calories total.

Breakfast in Meal Plan 5: 190 calories of potato pancakes Lunch: 290 calories of roast pork loin with garlic and rosemary

Dinner: 280 calories of peppercorn-sauteed salmon Sides/Snacks: 440 calories each of creamy spinach and cheesy cauliflower soup

One thousand two hundred calories total.

Meal Plan 6: Baked Beans for Breakfast, 250 Calories Nut-Crusted Chicken Breasts for Lunch, 320 Calories Dinner: 282 calories of slow-roasted pesto salmon

Gelatin with Peaches and Cottage Cheese + Creamy Chicken Vegetable Soup = 348 calories for sides/snacks.

One thousand two hundred calories total.

Meal Plan 7: Ground Pork Wonton Ravioli (130 calories) for breakfast Lunch: Rice and Curried Chicken Meatballs (210 calories).

Ranch-Seasoned Crispy Chicken Tenders for Dinner, 462 calories

Cream of Broccoli Soup with Turkey Bacon Brussels Sprouts (Sides/Snacks): 398 calories One thousand two hundred calories total.

CONCLUSION

Without a doubt, this diet is efficient, and it works wonders for weight loss. Ask for a calorie decrease to achieve a more balanced diet before starting the diet plan from your doctor, as well as the addition of any dietary supplements that truly contain nutrients that the body needs.

Given that it contains fewer calories than what your body needs each day, a diet of 1,200 calories per day is regarded as low-calorie.

Not even the greatest or the sole measure of general health is weight. It is actually not required for someone to merely lose weight in order to become healthier. In some situations, being underweight can actually be detrimental to one's health, especially if they consume unhealthy foods or don't obtain enough of the necessary elements in their diet.

A very low-calorie diet can also be difficult to follow, especially for people who already struggle to get enough food each day. Regardless of the type of weight loss a person chooses, it is crucial that they develop a diet and exercise program they can stick to for the rest of their lives.

Making a personalized diet and nutrition plan with the right balance of nutrient-dense meals and decadent foods may benefit from the help of a dietitian or nutritionist.